Keto Desserts:

The Easy to Follow Ketogenic Cookbook for your Low-Carb High-Fat Diet with 40 Fat Bombs And Sweet Snack Recipes. 2019 Edition

Amanda Jason

Table of Contents

Introduction

Congratulations on downloading your copy of the Keto Desserts: *The Easy to Follow Ketogenic Cookbook for your Low-Carb High-Fat Diet with 40 Fat Bombs and Sweet Snack Recipes.* I'm delighted that you have chosen to take this sweet avenue to incorporating the Keto diet plan in your life.

Whether you are new to the Keto diet or have been testing out the dishes for years, you will find the recipes; tricks and tips will help you prepare a healthy variety of sweets that will make your mouth water. The plan goes by many different names such as the low-carb diet, the Keto diet, and the low-carbohydrate diet & high-fat (LCHF) diet plan. However, we will keep it simple and call it the Keto diet in this cookbook.

Most of these recipes are quick and easy as we know that time is important to everybody. There are time and money saving tips inside that will help you to integrate the Kato diet pretty easily into your life. You will be able to make most of these recipes ahead of time and be able to store them for a quick snack when you need one and some dishes are ready to be served in less than 30 minutes!

There even is a section about the special tools that you can utilize in your kitchen. You might even find there will be some exciting additions to help you to make these recipes even more quickly.

Many of the recipes have a Tricks and Tips section that give you ideas on how to be creative with the recipes and experiment with your taste buds with these already superb sweeties. It is also an amazing opportunity to get the family in the kitchen with you to help and to learn about how to have a healthy relationship with food.

Some of the recipe items may require a few more steps, but each recipe will provide you with an estimated preparation and cooking time, amount of servings, and a list of nutritional values including calories, net carbohydrates, protein, and fats. It is all laid out for you in a simple to follow a list of instructions to get started on incorporating the Keto diet in your life today.

There are plenty of books on Keto diet in the market today and thanks again for choosing this one! Every effort was made to ensure that it is full of as much useful information as possible.

Chapter 1: Ingredients, Keto Dessert Essentials, and Tools you Need for Your Keto Desserts

Ingredients

There are some main ingredients that are an absolute necessity in the Keto diet to have the high-fat content that you need instead of the carbs. You will find these ingredients will be the new staple in your pantry, and here you will find out why these substitutes for your normal diet will not leave you dissatisfied. In fact, your body will thank you.

Butters

Almond butter in its pure form is simply ground roasted or raw almonds. It is a much healthier alternative to regular butter as there are no additives like sugar and it has 3 grams of net carbohydrates per serving.

However, you will find that there are different qualities out there. As such, while you are shopping, you must keep a sharp eye out for the ingredients lists and there can be many additives included that you did not expect.

To avoid this, stick with the almond butter that only has 6 total ingredients on the label. But do not stop there. Make sure there are no added oils as this is typical for the lesser quality almond butter. A good tip is to find an organic almond butter as they will not roast the raw almonds in vegetable oil and will typically just add salt for flavoring.

Cashew butter is a substitute for traditional butters that gives your dishes a sweet flavor naturally. It also helps your sweet treats to have a more rich and creamy dough. You may choose between 100% cashew butter or some varieties have sunflower oil included. Note that the butter with sunflower oil will add a more oily consistency to your sweet recipes, and they will be denser.

Coconut butter can be used as a substitute in these recipes instead of butter. This is a good choice for people who have lactose intolerance or a dairy allergy.

However, there are many health benefits to consuming coconut butter including antibacterial lauric acid. This will keep you feeling better inside and out as it especially wards off viral diseases of many varieties including yeast infections to bronchitis. It also contains medium-chain fatty acids that treat major diseases including diabetes and cancer. And, it is high in fiber and iron to boot! Consider changing to this healthy alternative in all your Keto recipes.

Grass-fed butter has been shown to have higher contents of nutrients such as linoleic acid (CLA) and loaded with beneficial fats and vitamins versus traditional butter, which generally comes from

GMO fed cows. Grass-fed butter also contains a dominant anti-inflammatory fat called butyric acid and anti-oxidants, which aid in your overall health.

Hazelnut butter is another healthy alternative to regular butter as it is high in vitamin E and manganese. You will find the more you research into the Keto diet that manganese is essential in aiding in fat and carb metabolism. This is exactly the super ingredient you have been looking for! As with all nut butters, the quality can differ. So be sure to read the ingredients list, and the best bet is to stick to the organic raw hazelnuts and shy away from added oils.

Flours

Almond flour is quite popular in the Keto diet as the main substitute for the traditional wheat flours. It has a much higher fat content than wheat flour, which tends to burn recipes much quicker. You will find that many of the oven temperatures in these recipes are lower than the traditional recipes for that very reason.

Because almond flour is made just from almonds, you can make it right in your kitchen. All you would need is a high powered blender to pulverize the almonds. The benefits with almond flour is that it is filled with heart-healthy fats and is naturally gluten-free, making it the number one choice in the Kato diet.

There are many other benefits to almond flour that will make you fall in love with it while you get acquainted with the Keto diet. It has been shown to manage healthy levels of blood sugar along with improving heart health. Improving energy levels and helping with weight loss, you cannot deny that almond flour is going to become your new pal in the kitchen.

As a rule of thumb, when you are converting old-fashioned recipes, you should use 50% more almond flour versus the amount of traditional wheat flour.

Coconut flour has extremely high levels of saturated fats (which are healthy for you!), and these fats actually aid in metabolism and assist in balancing out the blood sugar levels naturally. Coconut flour has many other benefits such as being low in sugar and carbs, high in fiber, and is absolutely packed with vitamins and minerals.

Even though it is more expensive (See Chapter 3 for the money saving tips!), it does not take much of this flour to go a long way in these recipes. There are smaller amounts needed for the Keto diet recipes compared to almond flour, as it is much more absorbent, and it fills you up more than traditional wheat flour. Because coconut flour is more absorbent, you will find those recipes will require more butter and eggs. The taste of the coconut flour also compliments many fruity dishes as well.

The reason why everyone loves coconut flour is because it aids your body to maintain healthy blood sugar levels and keeps them more stable. And as we said, it makes you feel fuller, so you will not be wanting to grab unneeded snacks during the day. Although you still may want to after seeing the treats we have in store for you!

Coconut flour actually improves digestive health, as well as keeping everything working on a regular cycle. This is due to it having five times more fiber as compared to the fiber levels in traditional wheat flour.

The metabolism benefits for coconut flour also offer quick energy as it contains medium-chain fatty acids (MCTs). These are healthy fats that help you to get up and going to keep burning off the fat.

And the benefits of coconut flour continues. It actually keeps you healthier by protecting your body because of the antiviral and antibacterial properties it contains. And, if you have a nut allergy, coconut flour is your best friend as you can use it for all of your baking needs without the worry of an allergic reaction.

Sweeteners

There is a wide variety of sweeteners available for Keto diet followers. We use Swerve throughout the book for most of the recipes because it is one of the top approved brands of sweetener for the Keto diet. It is also sugar-free! However, it is up to personal preference which sweetener you use.

Monks fruit sweetener is also a popular choice, you must know that this sweetener will make your dishes sweeter versus the other choices of sweeteners. However, the people who do prefer monks fruit sweetener find that other sweeteners have a cooling effect and bad aftertaste. If you find this to be true, this will be the choice in sweeteners for you.

Natvia icing mix is a combination of stevia and erythritol sweeteners resulting in the perfect icing that you are used to in old-fashioned recipes. But it is even better! It does not contain any artificial flavors or colors and does not cause plaque build-up on your teeth. Alternatively, you can use **Swerve Icing Sugar Style** in the recipes if you prefer the taste.

Sukrin Gold brown sugar substitute is also used by monks fruit lovers as it packs the same sweet taste. This can be used as a substitute for your Keto baking needs as it does not burn as hot as the other sweeteners and still has only 8 calories per hundred grams.

Stevia liquid drops can be used in many sweets and can be substituted particularly for the confectioner sweetener. It also contains no calories or carbs and does not alter your blood sugar levels. With over a dozen flavors to choose from, it can be the next must have to have section in your pantry.

Swerve has the same amount of sweetness compared to traditional white sugars found in recipes. It measures out to be the same if converting recipes after you get deeper into the world of Keto, as you will find yourself going through your grandmother´s recipes to convert them. There is also no calories in this sweetener, so it will help you to not feel guilty when you are eating those Keto cookies.

Truvia is the brand name for the natural sweetener of the stevia plant. Most people who are into eating healthy have heard of stevia or the common name is erythritol. This is a sugar alcohol that is found in melons and grapes and also has no calories. Many people say that there is a metallic taste to stevia, but others compare it to the same taste as traditional sugar. Again, experiment with the sweeteners to find what suits your palate.

As a note, if you have been diagnosed with autoimmune disorders or a leaky gut, Truvia may actually have ill effects for your digestive system. If you suffer from these disorders or are allergic to corn, consult your doctor about which sweetener is best for your personal diet.

You can use granulated sweeteners in place of confectioner sweeteners. If you do substitute the granulated sweeteners, you will find that you will be able to feel the texture of the granules in your sweet treats.

Also, the confectioner sweeteners will have a sweeter taste, so if you prefer less sweet, stay with the granulated sweetener. The confectioner sweeteners do work best in the sweet recipes, but it up to your personal preference.

Other Essentials

Agar agar is based on red algae. Gelatin can be used as an alternative, but it will not have the same consistency. When you use agar agar, you will get a more firm texture compared to gelatin and has more health benefits than gelatin. It is low in carbs, sugar, and calories and suppresses the appetite, making them great treats to have when your stomach rumbles.

9

Fresh organic eggs are recommended versus the eggs you buy in the carton from your grocery store. This is due to them usually containing MSG, and the packaging companies are not required to label this on the packaging. If you want to stay true to the Keto lifestyle, switch to the fresh organic egg option.

Organic eggs are high in phosphatidylcholine, which keeps the nervous system in the brain functioning at optimal levels. They are also high in protein, anti-oxidants, and vitamin E so you really cannot go wrong when you make the switch.

MCT oil is an abbreviation for the fats called medium chain triglycerides. You will find high counts of these fats in coconut oil. However, MCT oil is a more potent version compared to coconut oil alone. It is an excellent aid in losing weight as it burns more calories than it contains and it boosts your energy levels.

Mascarpone cheese comes from Italy and you will find it in the mousse recipes. You know, or will find out, that fatty cheeses are brilliant on the Keto diet, and this one does not disappoint. Because of the high-fat content, it has a more creamy consistency than cream cheese and a bonus is that the carb count is low as well.

Xanthan gum is used in particular with the cookie recipes to keep the cookies from crumbling, and it actually makes the cookies softer and tastier. It is usually an optional ingredient, but experiment with this ingredient, and you may find that you cannot live without it.

Keto Dessert Essentials

There are many tips in helping you with these recipes and others that you find along your journey into the Keto diet. Here are some basic cooking tips for this cookbook that you will find helpful for the different types of recipes.

Cookies

If you prefer to have crispy cookies while you try out these Keto diet delights, be sure to make sure to **let the cookies cool completely**, even if this means overnight. They will be less crumbly and you will not regret every crunch in your mouth.

If you prefer sweeter cookies, add 1/4 teaspoon **stevia glycerite** to any of the recipes to appease your sweet tooth.

If you find that you are not getting the fluffiness that you desire in your cookies, add 1/2 teaspoon of **apple cider vinegar** to the ingredients. It will alter the cookie texture, but it will give the cookies more rise.

Cakes

When you are **frosting the cakes**, be sure to make sure that the frosting is not applied to the cake while it is still warm. This will ensure that the frosting will not melt off as you are spreading it onto the cake.

You will find a **sprinkle** recipe that is based with coconut flakes. You can use this recipe to top any of your sweet treat desserts and it is brilliant for any occasion.

If you dread **cutting a cake** into uniform pieces, there are cake markers and cutters that you can buy that will save you the hassle. Most come in 14 or 16 slices.

Mousses

Of the recipes that are served right away without the use of the freezer or fridge, they are going to be more of the soft serve consistency. If you prefer to have a **more thick mousse**, simply put it in the fridge or freezer to harden it up.

Frozen Desserts

You will find that many of the desserts can be transformed into other sweet frozen treats. Keep an eye out for the Tricks and Tips at the end of the recipes for tips on how to add variety or other uses for the same recipes. You will find that you can get really creative with the recipes and still stay within the Keto diet guidelines.

Tools You Need

You will have many of these cooking utensils in your kitchen already, but if you collect these tools ahead of time, it will save you time, and you will have what you need to make the Keto diet a lifestyle change for you.

The items that you will need that you probably already own are the absolute basics for cooking and baking. These include basic **mixing dishes, electrical beater, stirring spoons, rolling pin**, **rubber scraper, fine mesh strainer,** and a **whisk**.

If you already do not own a **food processor** or a **high powered blender**, you will find these will be fantastic additions to your kitchen, as these will help you to be able to bake these recipes much more quickly compared to mixing ingredients by hand. This will also leave you able to do other methods or tell the children to do their homework in the meantime.

When you are baking sweet treats in the Keto diet, it is best to use **baking paper** or **silicone based pans and cooking trays** because they tend to stick to the pan more so than traditional recipes. The silicone products are brilliant when it comes to baking and especially with the Keto diet, as nothing will stick to the silicone. If you choose to use the parchment paper liners, they also have the benefit of sweeties not getting too wet on the bottom.

The **Silpat** or **non-stick mat** will make your life so much grander when it comes to keeping it simple with cleanup for the sweeties. It is easy to wash and nothing sticks to it. It is a good substitute for parchment paper, and it is reusable. The only downside is you cannot use sharp objects on the Silpat, as it will cause it damage.

Cookie scoopers are a nice addition to the collection, as I can guarantee you will be using this tool a lot after tasting these recipes. It will help to keep your cookies in a uniform shape and makes baking much easier than scraping the dough off a spoon.

For the cakes, you can use a **springform pan** to release the baked loaf without a bunch of fuss. It is used specifically in the *Birthday Cake Recipe* but you will find that you will need it when you gather even more recipes or convert your grandma´s cheesecake recipe.

If you are not familiar with springform pans, they come in two parts and are kept together by a spring lock mechanism. When you release the lock, the cake comes out rather easily, making these cake recipes a breeze.

You will find that many of these dishes you will want them to look like they came out of the bakery down the street. Many of the mousse and cake recipes call for having a **pastry bag**. You can find these in craft or baking good stores or you can fashion one yourself rather quickly using a ziplock bag.

This will be a way to decorate and pipe the ingredients into serving dishes that is a lot more beautiful than just spooning the dishes in by hand. Although, these sweet dishes might not even make it out of the mixing bowl!

All **ovens** heat differently depending on if they are along an outside wall of your home. Keep this in mind, as you may need to raise or lower the oven temperature up or down by 25° Fahrenheit to get the desired time of baking.

Chapter 2: Time and Money Saving Tips

In this day in age, we are always lacking in time and money. Well, the good news is many of these recipes are quick and easy. You will not need to spend all day in the kitchen struggling to make a healthy meal for yourself and your family. In fact, this is probably going to change the more you get involved in the Keto diet lifestyle as you start seeing how your body looks healthier and you will feel it in your mind as well.

Time Saving Tips

The biggest time-saving tip is you can double or even triple these recipes as they all keep for many days either on the counter or an even longer time in your freezer or refrigerator. It can't get easier than that!

You will find that the unfrosted cakes can be kept in the freezer for up to 3 months. When you are ready to use them, simply move them from the freezer to the fridge the day before you want to serve the cake. This will give the cake time to thaw properly and it will be a breeze to apply the frosting as well.

You can even keep the cakes in the refrigerator for up to a week before they will need to be eaten. Although, we would be surprised if they lasted that long!

If you are going to store your sweeties on the counter, keep them in an air-tight container as they will keep longer. As with the cookies, you can always keep them in the all familiar cookie jar as you know this always brings back wonderful memories of childhood. This method will also keep your sweet treats even softer. Most cookies will need to be eaten within 5 days if stored on the counter.

Storing your Keto sweets in the freezer or the refrigerator are just as easy. Simply wrap each pastry securely in plastic wrap, put them in a sealed container (only if putting into the refrigerator), or throw them into a zip-lock plastic bag. If you are storing them in the freezer, be sure to put them in a freezer safe container or zip lock bag.

Whenever you need to eat them, you can put them back into the oven to heat them up, throw them into the microwave, or even eat them straight out of the bag. This will make the cookies, in particular, crispier, as you have already learned. All other specific tips for the recipes will be found under the Tricks and Tips at the end of the recipe.

If you keep your sweeties in the fridge, they will keep for a week, and in the freezer, they will keep up to one month´s time.

The key before storing them away is to make sure that the sweets are completely cool beforehand. This will ensure that they will not end up crumbling to pieces and the excess moisture from the heat will not cause condensation on the packaging.

One tip to use for any of the baked goods using a pan, melt 2 teaspoons of coconut oil and brush the inside of the pan. Freeze for at least 20 minutes for the coconut oil to harden, and this will ensure the baked goods do not stick. This will come in handy as many of the recipes in Keto stick to the pan due to the alternative ingredients used.

Another time-saving tip is to get the family involved. It is a lost tradition to have the children or spouse help in the kitchen, but we guarantee that they will love to help! Simply even having them help you collect the ingredients that you will need will save time, and the kids will be learning some great life lessons by solidifying their cooking skills in the kitchen. And you will also be giving them the building blocks they need to live a healthier life as they grow up.

So do not feel the pressure of doing it all yourself. Even though many of these recipes are easy to do on your own, maybe consider letting the children make simple ones and work together with them on the more complex recipes. This will also help you have a closer relationship with your family as you will be able to spend more time with them.

Money Saving Tips

You will find that the ingredients that are called for in the Keto diet recipes are going to be more expensive. Mentally you will need to get past this fact because, again, you need to keep in mind why you have made the choice to begin this lifestyle change. Once you start seeing the benefits to your health, you will be hooked and try to find more ways to further your journey into this lifestyle change you have chosen.

Luckily, there are ways to ensure that you get the best bang for your buck when it comes to buying ingredients to stock your pantry. You will also find benefit in talking and researching on your own with what other people have found during their own personal journeys that it will help you on your own path. If this seems overwhelming at first, just take a deep breath. We have some good tips for you to follow making this transition as easy as possible.

Be sure to shop around for the best prices and educate yourself on the prices of items so you know you are getting the best deal, but know that the quality may vary. Read through the ingredients to make sure there are no other additives that are not specific to the Keto diet and do not ever lose hope.

To make sure that you are not wasting money, look through your kitchen and pantry and see what you already have. Many times mason jars or cans get forgotten about or stuffed behind something that we rarely use. If you go through the pantry and get rid of all the sugary and processed foods, it will make this process easier. You can even donate the items that you are not going to be able to eat to the local food pantry, as this is another way to give back to the community.

Once you have an idea what you already have, then just make sure that you try to use these items first and do not buy more unless it is an item that you will use regularly. When you throw food out, it is the same as throwing money out with it.

A good rule of thumb when you are shopping for Keto on a budget is to stray away from the prepackaged items that are labeled specifically Keto. You will find that if you look for these same products or ingredients that they will be cheaper. This is because with the Keto diet growing in popularity, the marketing corporations are trying to cash in. Do not be fooled!

Most times these prepackaged and Keto labeled items can be made more cheaply in your kitchen and will not take that much time to make yourself. However, if you are able and you simply do not have the time, the pre-packed items are following the Keto diet. Just know that you will be spending more money for the convenience.

One way to cut down costs is to make the almond and coconuts flours in your own kitchen. As stated before, the almond flour can be made at home using a high powered blender and buying raw almonds. This will also ensure the freshness of the final product, and you will feel even more empowered in your continued journey into the Keto diet.

Buying the ingredient components in bulk will also cut down on costs. For example, instead of buying the cheese already shredded, compare the prices to buying a block of the same cheese and grating it yourself. The time that it takes to accomplish this is minimal, and your pocket will feel the difference.

Another tip is to look for the sale prices and utilize weekly coupons in the Sunday paper or the deals offered by the grocery stores. Most items can be packed and stored in your freezer for later. This is especially true for fruits and vegetables as they are cheaper when they are in season. If you educate yourself on the options out there, you will find there are many shortcuts that will not hurt your waistline and your wallet will be fatter.

Even looking for fruits, cheeses, milk, and eggs at the local farmers market is a great tip, as they are the mom and pop growers that rely on you to keep in business. They will even have organic and GMO-free options most likely and might have some of the specialty items that you need. So shop locally whenever possible as you will feel better all around inside and out for helping the local community to grow themselves.

For instance, when you purchase almond meal at the supermarket, it is going to be about $10 dollars for each pound. Do not fret! Many of these recipes call for smaller amounts compared to traditional recipes. Remember, a little bit goes a long way.

Alternatively, you can look on Amazon.com to have your ingredients delivered straight to your door without the hassle. You will find that the prices for the ingredients you use most will be cheaper even with the shipping. Remember though to make sure the ingredients are in line with your Keto lifestyle and know they will be much better than the food choices that you are accustomed to eating.

You can also look into other flour substitutes such as flax meal, which has better benefits compared to almond flour. First off is the cost, as it will usually run you about $4 a pound compared to $10 a pound for the almond flour.

Again, saving money on the Keto diet is all about education and knowing where to look. Be creative with the ingredients and find cheaper alternatives. Another suggestion is to buy almond meal rather than almond flour. This is an ingredient that is easily substituted for almond flour, and most recipes will have this ingredient.

Costs for the coconut flour are considerably cheaper than almond flour, and you end up using less in the recipes. You can find several brands of coconut flour that will average about $5 per pound. Again, if you take advantage of the online shopping networks, you will have them delivered straight to you without the hassle of driving to several supermarkets to find the best price for your budget.

If you do not have a nut allergy, these would also be a good addition to your pantry and would substitute for the almond or coconut flours in the recipes. You will find that these nut flours will cost about $4 a pound as well.

I know it may not seem like a money saving tip at first glance, but if you plan your meals out ahead of time and make a shopping list, you are more likely to buy what you need. This cuts down on food waste and helps you to stay on track with your diet. When you shop, stay away from the isles that have been tempting in the past and certainly refrain from shopping while you are hungry. Although, the more you get into the Keto diet, you will find that the hunger will not strike as much.

Even though we stress about the benefits of the specialty ingredients that are available on the Keto diet, do not feel pressured to buy specific items if they do not fit into your budget. Remember the end goal of you trying to better your health by making better food choices.

If you are used to eating a pack of cookies in the afternoon with your soft drink as a snack, you would now be eating a low carb, filling chocolate drizzled granola bar instead. It is all about baby steps. Do not feel pressured to jump straight in and mind what you are able to afford. Even having carton eggs from the grocery is a better meal for breakfast than a bowl of processed sugary cereal.

This next tip is actually a time and money saver. You can double any of these recipes or even save the leftovers for eating the next day or later. This will make sure that you do not have to cook for every snack or meal, and you will have time to make other sweeties if you prefer.

As you get more accustomed to your new lifestyle, you will find you will naturally spend less money. This is because even these sweet treats will leave you satisfied for longer so you do not have to keep buying food because you are having a sugar crash or craving. As the basis of the Keto diet is to pack up the healthy fats in your daily diet, you will find that the portions you will want to eat will be less as well. Since you will most likely have leftovers, couple this up with the time-saving tip of packaging leftovers to serve later. Purchasing a FoodSaver is something that will pay for itself over the long run, as it will keep your Keto foods and sweeties from getting freezer burn. It also saves space, as it is essentially a vacuum that sucks out the air from the ziplock or plastic bags that you use to store your leftovers. Just make sure that you label items so that you know they are still fresh when you take them out to thaw.

Chapter 3: Cookie Recipes

Almond Cinnamon Butter Cookies

Total Prep & Cooking Time: 25 minutes

Makes: 12 Cookies

Protein: 3 grams

Net Carbs: 1.2 grams

Fat: 13 grams

Calories: 196

What you need:

2 cups blanched almond flour

1 tsp. ground cinnamon

1/2 cup butter, softened

1 large egg

1/2 cup Swerve sweetener, granulated

1 tsp. vanilla extract, sugar-free

Steps:

1. Set the stove temperature at 350° Fahrenheit. Use a non-stick baking mat if available or layer baking paper on a regular sized cookie sheet.
2. In a big dish, whisk the almond flour and butter completely.
3. Combine the sweetener and egg making sure the mixture is not lumpy.
4. Then add the vanilla extract and cinnamon until incorporated.

5. Use a cookie scooper to spoon out a small amount and roll by hand into 1 inch balls. Transfer to the prepared cookie sheet.

6. Using a fork, press the cookies firmly, first horizontally and then vertically to create a crisscross pattern.

7. Heat for 12 - 15 minutes in the stove. Remove and place on the counter to cool before serving.

Butter Pecan Cookies

Total Prep& Cooking Time: 25 minutes

Makes: 10 Cookies

Protein: 3 grams

Net Carbs: 2.7 grams

Fat: 11 grams

Calories: 116

What you need:

1/2 cup Swerve sweetener, granulated

1/2 tsp. vanilla extract, sugar-free

1/2 cup butter, unsalted

1 3/4 cups almond flour, blanched

1/2 cup pecans, chopped and toasted

2 tbsp. coconut flour

1/2 tsp. salt

Steps:

1. The stove needs to be set to 325° Fahrenheit. Cover 2 regular sized cookie sheets with baking paper or you can use silicone baking mats instead.
2. Using a big dish, cream the sweetener, vanilla extract, and butter with an electrical beater awaiting the consistency to be fluffy.
3. Combine the almond flour and coconut flour to the mixture until incorporated.
4. Then carefully fold the pecans and salt into the batter.

5. Scoop out the dough with a spoon or cookie scooper. Create 1 inch balls of dough. Lightly press them approximately 2 inches from each other on the prepared cookie sheets.

6. Heat in the stove for 5 minutes and transfer the cookie sheet to the counter. Use a smooth bottomed glass to press each cookie about 1/4 inches thick.

7. Heat in the stove for another 12 minutes.

8. Leave them to set on the cookie pan for approximately 10 minutes for them to set properly.

Chocolate Brownie Cookies

Total Prep & Cooking Time: 25 minutes

Makes: 6 Cookies

Protein: 2 grams

Net Carbs: 1.3 grams

Fat: 8 grams

Calories: 122

What you need:

1/4 cup almond flour

1/3 cup monk fruit sweetener

2 tsp. cocoa powder, unsweetened

1/4 tsp. baking powder, gluten-free

2 tbsp. coconut oil

1 tsp. vanilla extract, sugar-free

4 oz. chocolate chips, sugar-free

1/4 cup pecans, chopped

1 large egg

1/4 tsp. salt

Steps:

1. Set your stove to 370° Fahrenheit. Set out a non-stick baking mat or cover a regular sized cookie sheet with baking paper.
2. Heat a saucepan to melt the chocolate chips and coconut oil until smooth.
3. In a regular dish, whip the sweetener and eggs until together.
4. Stir in the baking powder, vanilla extract and salt thoroughly.

5. Pour the melted chocolate into the batter.

6. Add the almond flour and stir with a large spoon for about 1 minute. The dough will have a runny consistency.

7. Carefully stir the pecans and cocoa powder into the dough until fully incorporated.

8. Use a cookie scoop to spoon out 6 cookies onto the prepared baking sheet, placing the cookies about 2 inches apart.

9. Heat for 10 – 12 minutes and move to the counter. Wait approximately 20 minutes before serving.

Tricks and Tips:

- If you prefer a brownie texture to the cookies, take the baking sheet out of the stove after 12 minutes.

- If you would like the taste of the cookies to have more chocolate flavor, add an additional 1/4 cup of chocolate chips when you fold the pecans into the batter.

Chocolate Chip Cookies

Total Prep & Cooking Time: 25 minutes

Makes: 12 Cookies

Protein: 5 grams

Net Carbs: 10 grams

Fat: 14 grams

Calories: 178

What you need:

1/2 tsp. apple cider vinegar

1/4 tsp. Stevia sweetener, confectioner

1/2 tsp. baking soda

1 cup butter, cashew

2 large eggs

1 cup chocolate chips, stevia-sweetened

1/2 tsp. vanilla extract, sugar-free

Steps:

1. Set the stove to heat at 350° Fahrenheit. Use a non-stick baking mat or line a regular sized cooking sheet with baking paper.
2. In a food processor on the medium setting, whip the eggs until smooth. Add the sweetener and baking soda until mixed.
3. Add the apple cider vinegar and vanilla extract and stir with a rubber scraper.
4. Finally, combine the butter to the batter and mix completely.

5. Use a cookie scooper to spoon the dough to the prepared flat pan approximately 2 inches away from each other.
6. Heat in the stove for 12 – 14 minutes and transfer the cookies to the counter for 10 minutes to cool before serving.

Cream Cheese Cookies

Total Prep & Cooking Time: 1 hour 25 minutes

Makes: 15 Cookies

Protein: 1 gram

Net Carbs: 1 gram

Fat: 8 grams

Calories: 91

What you need:

1/2 cup coconut flour

1/4 tsp. salt

1/2 tsp. baking powder, gluten-free

3 tbsp. cream cheese, softened

1/2 cup Swerve sweetener, granulated

1 large egg

1/2 cup butter, softened

1 tsp. vanilla extract, sugar-free

Steps:

1. Place a piece of baking paper to the side.
2. In a big dish, cream the sweetener, vanilla extract and cream cheese with an electrical beater until smooth. Add the butter and egg and stir until incorporated.
3. Finally, mix the almond flour, baking powder and salt to the mixture, making sure the batter is not lumpy.

4. Transfer the dough to the piece of baking paper and mold into a log. Crimp the sides of the paper securely and harden in the refrigerator for approximately 60 minutes.

5. Set the stove to the temperature of 350° Fahrenheit. Cover a regular sized cookie sheet with baking paper. Alternatively, use a non-stick baking mat.

6. Remove the firmed dough from the refrigerator and slice into half inch pieces.

7. Place on the prepared flat pan with approximately 2 inches space in between and heat in the stove for 15 - 18 minutes. When the cookies are done, they will be brown on the edges.

8. Cool the cookies on the counter for at least 10 minutes before serving.

Peanut Butter Cookies

Total Prep & Cooking Time: 20 minutes

Makes: 10 Cookies

Protein: 3 grams

Net Carbs: 2.5 grams

Fat: 6 grams

Calories: 82

What you need:

1/2 cup peanut butter

1 large egg

1/2 cup Swerve sweetener, confectioners

1/2 tsp. vanilla extract, sugar-free

Steps:

1. Set your stove to the temperature of 350° Fahrenheit. Layer a regular sized cookie sheet with baking paper. You can also use a non-stick baking mat.
2. In a regular dish, blend the egg, Swerve, peanut butter and vanilla extract with a large rubber scraper.
3. Scoop out 1 1/2 tablespoons of dough with a spoon and roll into small balls. Place them on the prepared cookie sheet or mat.
4. Press the cookie balls with a fork, first horizontally and then vertically to create a crisscross pattern.

5. Heat in the stove for 12 - 15 minutes and transfer to the counter.

6. Wait 10 minutes to serve and enjoy!

Tricks and Tips:

- If you want an extra afternoon boost, add in a large scoop of protein powder into your peanut butter cookies.

Snickerdoodles

Total Prep & Cooking Time: 25 minutes

Makes: 16 Cookies

Protein: 4 grams

Net Carbs: 1.8 grams

Fat: 13 grams

Calories: 139

What you need:

For the cookie dough:

1 1/2 cup almond flour

2 tsp. cream of tartar

1/2 cup coconut flour

3/4 cup monk fruit sweetener, granulated

1/2 cup butter

1 tsp. baking soda

2 large eggs

1 tsp. vanilla extract, sugar-free

2 tsp. ground cinnamon

1/2 tsp. xanthan gum

1/8 tsp. salt

For the coating:

2 tbsp. monk fruit sweetener, granulated

1 tsp. ground cinnamon

Steps:

1. Set the temperature of the stove to 350° Fahrenheit. Layer the regular sized cookie sheet with baking paper. Alternatively, use a non-stick baking mat.
2. In a big dish, whisk the almond flour and baking soda together until it is not lumpy.
3. Add the coconut flour, cinnamon, cream of tartar, xanthan gum and salt until combined together.
4. In an additional big dish, cream the sweetener, vanilla extract, butter and eggs and with an electrical beater. Slowly add in the flour, making sure incorporated thoroughly.
5. In a dish, blend the coating of sweetener and cinnamon.
6. Spoon out about 2 tablespoons of dough using a cookie scoop. Roll by hand into individual balls.
7. Liberally cover the dough balls in the bowl of coating until the dough is completely concealed.
8. Lightly press the cookies on the prepared cookie sheet.
9. Heat in the stove for 12 minutes and remove the baking sheet to the counter. Cool for 10 minutes before serving.

Sugar-Free Sugar Cookies

Total Prep & Cooking Time: 6 hours 25 minutes

Makes: 24 Cookies

Protein: 2 grams

Net Carbs: 0.8 grams

Fat: 5 grams

Calories: 59

What you need:

1 1/4 cups almond flour

1/2 tsp. baking powder, gluten-free

5 tbsp. butter

1/2 cup monk fruit sweetener, granulated

1 tsp. vanilla extract, sugar-free

1/2 tsp. almond extract

4 tbsp. coconut flour

1 large egg

1/4 tsp. salt

Steps:

1. Place a piece of saran wrap to the side.
2. In a big dish, cream the sweetener, vanilla extract, and butter with an electrical beater until smooth. Add the egg, baking powder, and almond extract until fluffy and light.
3. Stir in the almond flour, salt and coconut flour with a rubber scraper.

4. Transfer the dough to the saran wrap, roll into a large ball and wrap tightly.

5. Refrigerate the wrapped dough for a least 6 hours. Alternatively, it can be left overnight.

6. After the dough is firm, make sure your stove is set at 375 ° Fahrenheit. Use a non-stick baking mat or cover a regular sized cookie sheet with baking paper.

7. Using 2 pieces of baking paper, place the chilled dough in between them and roll to approximately 1/4 inch thick.

8. Use the size and shape of cookie cutters that you prefer and cut the dough. Transfer the cut cookies to the prepared cookie sheet using a large spatula.

9. Heat in the stove for 10 – 11 minutes until golden. Remove the sheet to the counter. Wait 10 minutes for the cookies to cool before serving.

Chapter 4: Cake Recipes

Birthday Cake

Total Prep & Cooking Time: 1 hour 45 minutes + 3 hours 40 minutes
with sprinkles

Yields: 16 Slices

Protein: 6 grams

Net Carbs: 3.2 grams

Fat: 21 grams

Calories: 282

What you need:

For the cake:

40 drops Stevia drops, vanilla flavored

1/4 cup coconut flour

1 3/4 cup Swerve sweetener, granulated

1 cup almond flour

3 large eggs

1 tsp. baking powder, gluten-free

4 tbsp. coconut milk

Coconut oil cooking spray

16 tbsp. coconut oil

1 tsp. vanilla extract, sugar-free

1 tsp. maple extract

1/2 tsp. salt

For the frosting:

2 medium avocados, peeled

1/2 tsp. salt

2 oz. dark chocolate, unsweetened

3/4 cup Swerve sweetener, confectioner

1/2 tsp. maple extract

22 drops Stevia drops, vanilla flavored

For the sprinkles: *(optional)*

3-6 drops food coloring

8 oz. coconut, unsweetened and shredded

1 tsp. water

Steps:

Sprinkles:

1. Make the sprinkles the day before as they need to dry overnight. Prepare a cookie sheet with a piece of wax or baking paper.
2. Place 8 tablespoons of coconut in a dish. Add 3-6 drops of food coloring and 1 teaspoon of water. Stir until the coloring is what you desire, adding more food coloring or water if needed.
3. Transfer to the prepared cookie sheet and put in a place it will be undisturbed overnight so the coconut can dry.
4. Repeat the steps for additional colors, if you prefer.

Cake:

1. Note: the recipe ingredients above is only for one layer of cake. Double the recipe if you want a two layer cake.

2. Set your stove to be at the temperature of 350° Fahrenheit. Trim a circle of baking sheet to match the size of the springform pan.

3. Apply the cooking spray liberally inside and place the baking paper in the base of the pan. Spray additional cooking spray on top of the baking paper.

4. In a food processor on the setting of high, beat the sweetener, coconut oil, liquid stevia, and salt together for 30 seconds.

5. Add in the maple extract to the mixture.

6. Blend the coconut milk, vanilla extract, and eggs to the bowl and pulse for 30 seconds more.

7. Pour the almond and coconut flours for an additional 30 seconds. The mixture will have the consistency of dry cake batter at this point.

8. With a rubber scraper, carefully stir the rainbow sprinkles (optional) into the batter until incorporated.

9. Transfer the cake batter to the springform pan and heat for 35 minutes. Check with a toothpick to ensure the cake is baked fully in the middle.

10. Move the cake pan onto a cutting board. Wait for approximately 5 minutes and unlock the pan.

Frosting:

1. Heat a saucepan to melt the chocolate fully.

2. Using the food processor on the high setting, pulse the avocados and sweetener until smooth.

3. Add the liquid Stevia, maple extract and salt until combined.
4. For the desired consistency, you can add 1 teaspoon of water until the frosting thins. Be sure all ingredients are mixed thoroughly by scraping the sides between pulses.
5. Taste test the frosting and add additional sweetener if preferred.

Frosting the cake:

1. Ensure that the cake(s) has cooled completely before frosting.
2. Move the cake onto the center of a cake plate.
3. Start by frosting the middle of the top and finish with the sides.
4. If you have more than one layer, frost the middle of the first layer. Then stack the other cake above. Frost the top and then frost the sides.
5. Add more sprinkles on top of the cake, if desired and serve!

Tricks and Tips:

- The recipe for the frosting will also work for icing 12 cupcakes or can be put in a container with a lid in the refrigerator when ready to use.
- The cake can be frozen and defrosted in the refrigerator a day before you are ready to frost.
- The leftover sprinkles can be stored in a mason jar and placed in the pantry until the next celebration.

Carrot Cake

Total Prep & Cooking Time: 1 hour 50 minutes

Makes: 12 Slices

Protein: 7 grams

Net Carbs: 3.9 grams

Fat: 29 grams

Calories: 480

What you need:

For the cake:

1 cup Swerve sweetener, granulated

2 1/2 tsp. baking powder, gluten-free

1/2 cup Sukrin Gold brown sugar substitute

1 cup butter, unsalted and room temperature

2 1/2 cups almond flour, finely milled

1/2 cup coconut, unsweetened and flaked

2 cups grated carrots

1/2 cup heavy whipping cream

2 tsp. ground ginger

1 cup pecans, raw and roughly chopped

5 large eggs

1/2tsp. ground nutmeg

2 tbsp. cinnamon powder

1/2 tsp. salt

For the frosting:

3/4 cup heavy whipping cream

1 1/4 cup Swerve sweetener, confectioner

3/4 cup unsalted butter, softened

12 oz. cream cheese, full fat

For the topping:

1 cup pecans, raw and roughly chopped

Steps:

Cake:

1. Set your stove to the temperature of 350° Fahrenheit. Use cooking spray or heavily butter the sides and base of two 9 inch cake pans. Cover them with baking paper.
2. In a regular dish, blend the sweetener and butter until mixed well. Add 1 egg and beat into the mixture and repeat until all eggs are combined.
3. Stir the heavy whipping cream, brown sugar and carrots into the batter until thoroughly incorporated.
4. In a big dish, whisk the almond flour remove the lumps if present.
5. Then add the cinnamon powder, ground nutmeg, baking powder, and ground ginger.
6. Slowly combine the flour to the cake batter. Incorporate the coconut and pecans until mixed together.

7. Evenly distribute the batter in the prepared cake pans and heat in the stove for 35 minutes. Use a toothpick in the middle of the cake to make sure it is baked properly.

8. Remove to the counter and let it rest for 10 minutes. Unlock the pan and set the cake to the side until ready to frost.

Frosting:

1. Using a food processor on high, whisk the butter, sweetener and cream cheese for 3 minutes. Scrape the dish with a rubber scraper as necessary and continue to blend until fully incorporated.

2. Pour the heavy whipping cream into the frosting and beat for an additional 2 minutes until airy.

3. Move the first layer on a cake platter and apply the frosting to the top, keeping an even layer. Put the second cake above and apply frosting to the top.

4. Then frost the edges of the layers of cake keeping the frosting as even as possible.

5. Dust the top with the chopped pecans, cut into slices and serve.

Tricks and Tips:

• If you do not want to go through all the trouble of the layered cake, you can always use a 13 x 9 cake pan and add the frosting while the cake is still in the pan.

Chocolate Cake

Total Prep & Cooking Time: 10 hours 5 minutes

Makes: 12 Slices

Protein: 6 grams

Net Carbs: 2 grams

Fat: 18 grams

Calories: 19

What you need:

For the filling:

2 3/4 cup almond flour

1 1/2 cups sweetener, granulated

2 tsp. baking powder, gluten-free

1/2 cup butter, melted

4 oz. dark chocolate, stevia sweetened

1/2 cup cocoa powder, unsweetened

6 large eggs

1 avocado, pureed

2 tsp. vanilla extract, sugar-free

1 tsp. salt

For the icing:

1/2 cup butter

liquid stevia, to taste

1/2 cup cocoa powder, unsweetened

1/8 tsp. salt

Steps:

Cake:

1. Set your stove to the temperature of 350° Fahrenheit. Use cooking spray or heavily butter an 8-inch cake pan or cover with parchment lining.
2. In a regular dish, combine the eggs, avocado, baking powder, and vanilla extract until mixed well.
3. Add the almond flour, sweetener, dark chocolate and butter until incorporated. Then add the salt and cacao powder until smooth.
4. Distribute the cake batter into the prepped pan and heat in the stove for 45 minutes. Using a wooden stick, press it into the middle of the cake to make sure it is baked properly.
5. Transfer to the counter and remove from the pan. Set to the side.

Frosting:

1. Heat a saucepan to liquefy the butter completely.
2. Combine the cacao powder, salt, and liquid stevia and mix until smooth.
3. Let the icing completely cool before frosting the cake.
4. Remember to frost the middle first. Then to complete the frosting, down the sides.

Cinnamon & Nutmeg Cake

Total Prep & Cooking Time: 1 hour 55 minutes

Makes: 14 Slices

Protein: 7 grams

Net Carbs: 3 grams

Fat: 24 grams

Calories: 374

What you need:

For the cake:

1 1/2 cups almond flour

5 oz. butter, unsalted and softened

1 tsp. ground cinnamon

3/4 cup sweetener, granulated

1 tsp. baking powder, gluten-free

2 tbsp. coconut flour

1/2 tsp. ground ginger

5 oz. cream cheese, softened

1/4 tsp. ground cloves

1/2 tsp. ground nutmeg

5 large eggs

1/8 tsp. salt

For the icing:

2/3 cup Natvia icing mix

4 oz. butter, unsalted and softened

2 tbsp. heavy whipping cream

4 oz. cream cheese, softened

1 tsp. ground cinnamon

Steps:

Cake:

1. Set the temperature of the stove to 350° Fahrenheit. Use butter to liberally grease an 8-inch cake pan and place baking paper to cover the base of the cake pan.
2. In a big dish, blend the cream cheese and baking powder using an electrical beater.
3. Add the butter and sweetener until combined. Then sprinkle the cinnamon, cloves, nutmeg, and salt into the mixture.
4. Combine the almond flour, coconut flour, and eggs making sure there are no lumps present. Use a scraper on the dish and thoroughly mix.
5. Distribute the cake batter in the prepared pan and heat in the stove for 30 – 40 minutes. Ensure it is baked all the way through by poking a toothpick into the middle.
6. Remove the pan and place on the cake platter. Set to the side.

Frosting:

1. In a regular dish, blend cream cheese until the mixture is creamy.
2. Combine the butter and mix thoroughly.
3. Add the Natvia icing mix one spoonful at a time to ensure it gets completely mixed. Then combine the heavy whipping cream and cinnamon, continuing to stir the frosting until smooth.
4. Frost the middle first and then complete the frosting process after the cake has completely cooled.

Tricks and Tips:

- You can store this cake in the freezer for up to 3 months. Make sure it is wrapped tightly with plastic wrap or a freezer ziplock bag.

Coffee Cake

Total Prep & Cooking Time: 50 minutes

Makes: 12 Slices

Protein: 5.5 grams

Net Carbs: 1.7 grams

Fat: 22.9 grams

Calories: 320

What you need:

For the cake:

2/3 cup coconut flour

1 1/4 cup monk fruit sweetener, granulated

2/3 cup coconut oil, softened

1 tsp. baking soda

9 large eggs

1/2 tsp. ground cinnamon

2 tsp. vanilla extract, sugar-free

3/4 tsp. xanthan gum

1/2 tsp. salt

2 tsp. cream of tartar

For the topping:

3 tbsp. coconut flour

1/4 cup monk fruit sweetener, granulated

1 cup coconut, shredded

5 tbsp. coconut oil, melted

1 1/4 tsp. ground cinnamon

Steps:

1. Set your stove to the temperature of 350° Fahrenheit. Use butter to liberally lubricate a 9-inch square pan.
2. In a big dish, cream the eggs with an electrical beater. Add the coconut oil and vanilla extract mixing thoroughly.
3. In a separate dish, whisk the sweetener and coconut flour and blend until there are no lumps in the batter.
4. Add in the cinnamon, cream of tartar, xanthan gum and salt until incorporated.
5. Combine slowly all of the ingredients with an electrical beater until the dough forms.
6. Distribute the batter to the prepped cake pan and heat in the stove for 35 minutes.
7. In an additional dish, whisk the sweetener and coconut with an electrical beater until mixed together. Then stir in the coconut oil, cinnamon, and coconut flour until crumbly.
8. Pull the cake out of the stove and move to the counter for 30 minutes to cool in the pan.
9. Apply the crumble topping and slice before serving.

Tricks and Tips:

- Another tip to not have the cake stick to the pan is to brush 2 teaspoons of coconut oil that has been melted along inside of the pan. Put in the freezer until you are ready to bake.

- Take note that this recipe is a nut and dairy free, so feel free to enjoy this recipe with your morning coffee!

Cream & Berries Cake

Total Prep & Cooking Time: 1 hour 10 minutes

Makes: 8 Slices

Protein: 1 gram

Net Carbs: 5 grams

Fat: 22 grams

Calories: 236

What you need:

For the cake:

1 3/4 cup almond flour

2 tsp. baking powder, gluten-free

1 cup sweetener, granulated

2 tsp. vanilla extract, sugar-free

7 large eggs

1/2 tsp. cream of tartar

For the filling:

1 cup sweetener, granulated

8 oz. cream cheese, softened

2 cups mixed berries

1 tsp. vanilla extract, sugar-free

2 cups heavy whipping cream

1/2 cup raspberries

For the topping:

1 cup mixed berries

Steps:

10. Set your stove to the temperature of 350° Fahrenheit. Cover a jelly roll pan with baking paper or a non-stick mat.
11. In a food processor set on medium/high, cream the vanilla extract, eggs and cream of tartar for 9 minutes.
12. In a big dish, combine the almond flour and sweetener to remove all lumps. Add 1 egg and combine well. Repeat until all eggs are mixed.
13. Blend in the baking powder.
14. Use a rubber scraper to combine the whipped cream. It needs to keep the fluffiness while being incorporated into the batter.
15. Evenly distribute the cake batter in the prepared roll, coating to the edges with a rubber scraper. Heat in the stove for 20 – 22 minutes.
16. Place a tea towel on top of a wire rack. Straight after the cake is taken out of the stove, take a blunt edge to slice along the cake to make sure it is not stuck to the pan. Turn the cake upside down onto the tea towel and remove the pan.
17. Using the tea towel, roll the cake in a circle and tie the tea towel around it to keep it in place while it cools. Leave to the side while making the filling and whipped cream.
18. In the food processor set on medium, cream the vanilla extract, sweetener, and cream cheese until there are no lumps

present. Add in the raspberries and stir, crushing them into the batter.

19. In an additional bowl, cream the heavy whipping cream on high with an electrical beater for 4 minutes.

20. Use a rubber scraper to combine the cream cheese and whipping cream and beat again for 30 seconds.

21. Once the cake has cooled, carefully unroll to evenly distribute the filling over the entire cake. Shake the mixed berries on top of the filling and use the tea towel to roll back into place.

22. Put the rolled cake onto a serving plate and sprinkle the rest of the mixed berries on top. Slice and serve.

Lemon Pound Cake

Total Prep & Cooking Time: 1 hour 25 minutes

Makes: 16 Slices

Protein: 7 grams

Net Carbs: 3.4 grams

Fat: 22 grams

Calories: 255

What you need:

For the cake:

2 1/2 cups almond flour

1 tsp. lemon extract

8 oz. cream cheese

1 1/2 cups Swerve sweetener, confectioner

4 oz. butter

1 1/2 tsp. baking powder, gluten-free

8 large eggs

1 1/2 tsp. vanilla extract, sugar-free

1/2 tsp. salt

For the topping:

1/4 cup Swerve sweetener, confectioner

3 tbsp. heavy whipping cream

1/2 tsp. vanilla extract, sugar-free

Steps:

1. In a regular dish, combine sweetener with butter with an electrical beater until smooth. Add the cream cheese, baking powder and vanilla extract and continue to blend the mixture together.

2. Combine the eggs and lemon extract until the batter is incorporated.

3. Blend in the almond flour and salt, making sure no lumps are left in the batter.

4. Set your stove to the temperature of 350° Fahrenheit. Use butter to grease a regular sized cake pan.

5. Distribute the batter in the prepared cake pan and heat in the stove for 60 minutes. Stick a toothpick into the middle to ensure it is thoroughly baked.

6. While the cake is in the stove, use a regular dish to blend the sweetener, vanilla extract, and heavy whipping cream and use an electrical beater to combine until creamy.

7. Remove the cake pan to the counter for 30 minutes to cool before putting the frosting on top.

Vanilla Cake

Total Prep & Cooking Time: 45 minutes

Makes: 8 Slices

Protein: 3 grams

Net Carbs: 3.4 grams

Fat: 22 grams

Calories: 229

What you need:

For the cake:

1/4 cup coconut oil

3 tbsp. Swerve sweetener, granulated

1/4 cup coconut flour, sifted

1/8 tsp. salt

2 tsp. vanilla extract, sugar-free

1/4 tsp. baking soda

4 large eggs, separated

1 tsp. cream of tartar

For the frosting:

1 cup Swerve sweetener, confectioner

1/2 cup butter, unsalted

2 tbsp. heavy whipping cream

1 tsp. vanilla extract, sugar-free

Steps:

1. Set your stove to the temperature of 350° Fahrenheit. Use coconut oil to grease a 6-inch cake pan or use baking paper to cover the pan.
2. In a big dish, cream the egg whites with an electrical beater for 4 minutes. Blend in the cream of tartar and set to the side.
3. In a regular dish, whip the egg yolks and coconut oil until combined.
4. Add the coconut flour and baking soda and mix thoroughly.
5. Finally, add the sweetener, vanilla extract, and salt until completely blended.
6. Carefully fold the egg whites in small amounts to ensure they do not lose their fluffiness.
7. Distribute to the prepped cake pan and heat in the stove for 20 minutes. Stick a toothpick into the cake to ensure it is thoroughly baked.
8. While the cake is in the stove, use a regular sized dish to make the frosting. Whip the butter with the electrical beater and add the sweetener in small amounts until fully mixed.
9. Finally, add the vanilla extract and heavy cream and blend until the batter is smooth.
10. Move the baked caked to the counter for 30 minutes to cool before applying the frosting on the cake.

Tricks and Tips:

- If you want to use a standard 8 or 9-inch pan, just double the recipe.

Chapter 5: Tart and Bar Recipes

Tart Recipes

Butter Tarts

Total Prep & Cooking Time: 1 hour

Makes: 24 Tarts

Protein: 3 grams

Net Carbs: 6.9 grams

Fat: 14 grams

Calories: 174

What you need:

For the crust:

1/8 tsp. salt

1/4 cup sweetener, granulated

1 cup butter

2 cups almond flour

For the filling:

3 tbsp. almond flour

1/4 cup butter

1 tbsp. baking powder, gluten-free

3 large eggs, beaten

1 tsp. vanilla extract, sugar-free

1 1/4 cups Sukrin Gold brown sugar substitute

3/4 cup coconut, unsweetened

1/8 tsp. salt

Steps:

1. Set your oven to the temperature of 350° Fahrenheit. Heavily coat a 13 x 9 baking pan with butter.
2. In a big dish, mix the sweetener and butter with an electrical beater until combined. Then blend the almond flour and salt to the mixture until soft.
3. Distribute the dough to the prepared baking pan and spread evenly.
4. Use an additional big dish to cream the butter with an electrical beater until fluffy. Blend the eggs, brown sugar substitute, and vanilla extract and whip until combined.
5. Add the almond flour and salt to the mixture and combine thoroughly. Fold in the coconut and baking powder with a rubber scraper until totally incorporated.
6. Pour the filling over the dough in the prepared baking pan.
7. Heat in the stove for 30 - 35 minutes.
8. Move to cool on the counter completely before cutting into squares.

Blueberry Lemon Tarts

Total Prep & Cooking Time: 1 hour
Makes: 4 Tarts
Protein: 8 grams
Net Carbs: 4.9 grams
Fat: 20 grams
Calories: 21

What you need:

For the crust:

1/4tsp. monk fruit sweetener
2 tbsp. coconut oil, melted
1/4 cup coconut flour
2 1/2 cups pecan pieces, raw
1/8tsp. salt
2 tbsp. almond butter, smooth

For the filling:

3/4 cup lemon juice
12 tbsp. butter, unsalted and cubed
4 large eggs
1/4 cup lemon zest
2 tsp. monk fruit sweetener
1/8tsp. salt

For the topping:

2 cups blueberries

Steps:

Crust:

1. Liberally butter four 4 3 /4-inch tart pans or cover with baking paper.
2. Use a food blender to combine the coconut flour, coconut oil, and almond butter for 2 minutes on high.
3. Add the monk fruit, pecan pieces, and salt until crumbly.
4. Dividing the batter into 4 equal parts, transfer them to the tart pans. Evenly compress the crust by hand. Begin with the sides of the pan with the middle being pressed last. Put in the refrigerator to set.

Filling:

1. In a regular dish, blend together the sweetener and lemon zest and stir with a large spoon.
2. Heat a medium saucepan halfway filled with water on low/medium.
3. In a heatproof big dish, pour in the lemon juice, lemon zest, and eggs. Place the bowl on top of the saucepan.
4. Wait until the water starts to simmer. Then whisk the ingredients until they thicken for approximately 10 minutes.

5. Using a fine-mesh strainer, pour and press the curd into a blender.

6. After adding the salt, turn the blender on the low setting. Start adding the cubes of butter 3 pieces at a time and repeat until all the butter is blended.

7. Move the tart pans to the counter and pour the filling inside the crusts.

8. Put the tart pans back into the refrigerator for 20 minutes to set and cool.

9. Shake the blueberries over the tarts and serve.

Tricks and Tips:

- If you prefer your crust baked, put the tart pans in the stove at 375° Fahrenheit. Heat the crusts for 13 minutes. Then follow steps 7 through 9.

- If not eating the curd right away, pour into a container with plastic wrap tightly pressed on the top. Keep in the fridge, and the curd will stay fresh for 1 week.

Fruit and Cheese Tarts

Total Prep & Cooking Time: 2 hours 15 minutes

Makes: 12 Tarts

Protein: 5 grams

Net Carbs: 5 grams

Fat: 16 grams

Calories: 187

What you need:

12 prepared tart crusts, (see tricks and tips below)

1/3 cup lemon juice

14 oz. condensed milk, sweetened

1 tsp. lemon zest

8 oz. cream cheese, softened

1/4 cup crab apple jelly, melted

3 tbsp. coconut, toasted

12 pineapple chunks

1 tsp. almond extract

12 blackberries

4 large strawberries, sliced

1 tsp. vanilla extract, sugar-free

Steps:

1. Place the prepared tart crusts on two baking paper lined cookie sheets. You can also use a non-stick baking mat.

2. In a regular dish, blend together the cream cheese and condensed milk until soft. Combine the lemon zest and lemon juice, stirring with a rubber scraper. Then blend the almond extract and vanilla extract until smooth.

3. Sprinkle 4 teaspoons of toasted coconut into each tart crust and pour the cream cheese on top.

4. Put the tarts into the refrigerator for 2 hours to harden.

5. Just before serving, use a small saucepan on low heat to melt the crab apple jelly.

6. Remove the tarts and garnish with a strawberry slice, pineapple chunk, and a blackberry. Drizzle the crab apple jelly on top of the fruit and serve.

Tricks and Tips:

•   If you prefer your crust to be homemade, follow the baked tart crust steps in the *Blueberry Lemon Tart* recipe.

Hazelnut Tarts

Total Prep & Cooking Time: 2 hours 20 minutes

Makes: 8 Tarts

Protein: 6 grams

Net Carbs: 3 grams

Fat: 18 grams

Calories: 223

What you need:

2 tbsp. coconut oil, melted

4 prepared tart crusts, baked (see tricks and tips below)

1/4 cup butter, hazelnut and melted

2 tbsp. coconut cream, melted

1 tbsp. sweetener, granulated

2 oz. chocolate, unsweetened and melted

Steps:

1. Put the tart crusts on a baking pan covered with a non-stick mat or baking paper.
2. Heat a saucepan to melt the coconut cream and chocolate on until smooth. Stir in the sweetener and butter until combined.
3. In a separate small saucepan, melt the hazelnut butter until there are no lumps.
4. Measure out 1 tablespoon of melted butter and put in a tart crust. Repeat for all servings.
5. Then distribute the chocolate mixture evenly to each tart crust.

6. Place in the refrigerator for 2 hours to completely set.

Tricks and Tips:

- If you prefer your crust to be homemade, follow the baked tart crust steps in the Blueberry Lemon Tart recipe.
- Hazelnut butter not available in your local grocery? You can substitute with another nut butter of your choice. Almond butter is a good choice for this recipe.
- Having a hard time finding coconut cream? Just chill some coconut milk overnight and skim the cream that is on the top of the milk.
- If you love the taste of coconut, try adding some toasted coconut on the top before serving.
- For a variety in flavors, add some orange or ginger extract to the batter for some extra zing.

Bar Recipes

Chocolate Fudge Bars

Total Prep & Cooking Time: 15 minutes

Makes: 16 Bars

Protein: 3 grams

Net Carbs: 8.1 grams

Fat: 8 grams

Calories: 114

What you need:

8 oz. chocolate chips, unsweetened

1/2 cup peanut butter

Steps:

1. Cover an 8 square inch pan with baking lining and set to the side.
2. Heat a saucepan to melt the chocolate chips until liquefied. Then blend in the peanut butter until the batter is smooth.
3. Distribute to the prepped pan and level out with a rubber scraper
4. Put the fudge into the freezer for 10 minutes to firm.
5. Slice and enjoy!

Tricks and Tips:

- If you have an allergy to peanuts, you can substitute coconut butter, almond butter or sun butter instead.
- There are many varieties that you can experiment with by adding your favorite ingredients. Try shredded coconut, chopped walnuts or chia seeds.

Granola Bars

Total Prep& Cooking Time: 30 minutes

Makes: 8 Bars

Protein: 8 grams

Net Carbs: 2.8 grams

Fat: 28 grams

Calories: 306

What you need:

For the granola:

1/3 cup monk fruit sweetener

2 tsp. vanilla extract, sugar-free

1/4 cup coconut oil

1/2 cup almonds, sliced

1/4 cup coconut, unsweetened and shredded

1/3 cup flaxseed meal

1/2 cup almond butter, smooth

1/3 cup pumpkin seeds, shelled

1 tbsp. chia seeds

1/2 tsp. ground cinnamon

For the drizzle:

1 tsp. coconut oil

3 tbsp. dark chocolate chips, sugar-free

For the topping:

1 tbsp. almonds, sliced

Steps:

1. Using a regular loaf pan, layer with baking paper and set to the side.
2. Heat a pot to liquefy the sweetener, coconut oil, almond butter, and vanilla extract.
3. In a big dish, combine the almonds and coconut with a rubber scraper. Then add the flaxseed meal, pumpkin seeds, chia seeds, and cinnamon to fully incorporate.
4. Transfer the granola to the prepared pan and press down the mixture by hand to make uniform.
5. Freeze the granola for 20 minutes to harden.
6. In a saucepan, dissolve the chocolate chips and coconut oil together.
7. When set, remove and move the granola onto a serving plate.
8. Dust the almonds on the top and drizzle the chocolate over the almonds. Freeze for 3 additional minutes.
9. Cut into 8 individual bars and enjoy!

Tricks and Tips:

- These granola bars can be individually wrapped in plastic wrap and are perfect for on the go snacks. They will keep for up to 8 days in the refrigerator.

- Instead of putting the granola in the freezer, you can leave it in the refrigerator overnight to set and complete steps 7 through 9.

Lemon Bars

Total Prep & Cooking Time: 1 hour

Makes: 8 Bars

Protein: 8 grams

Net Carbs: 4 grams

Fat: 26 grams

Calories: 272

What you need:

1 cup sweetener, confectioner

3 large eggs

1/4 tsp. salt

1 3/4 cups almond flour

3 medium lemons

1/2 cup butter, melted

Steps:

5. Set your stove to the temperature of 350° Fahrenheit. Cover an 8-inch cake pan with baking paper and set to the side.

6. In a big dish, blend 1 cup of the almond flour and butter until fully incorporated. Add the sweetener (1/4 cup) and salt (1/8 teaspoon) and combine completely.

7. Push the batter squarely into the prepped pan and heat for 20 minutes. Remove and set on a heat resistant surface while mixing the filling.

8. Zest 1 lemon in a dish and add the juice from all 3 lemons. Add the remaining 3/4 cup almond flour and mix well.

9. Add 1 egg and cream into the mixture, repeating for all the eggs.

10. Finally, add the sweetener (3/4 cup) and salt (1/8 teaspoon) and incorporate thoroughly.

11. Transfer the filling to the cooled baking pan and heat in the stove for 25 more minutes.

12. Remove and dust the top with sweetener and garnish with a slice of lemon, if preferred.

Peanut Butter Chocolate Bars

Total Prep & Cooking Time: 2 hours 10 minutes

Makes: 8 Bars

Protein: 7 grams

Net Carbs: 4 grams

Fat: 8 grams

Calories: 246

What you need:

For the bars:

1/2 cup peanut butter

3/4 cup almond flour

1/4 cup Swerve Icing Sugar Style

2 oz. butter

1/2 tsp. vanilla extract, sugar-free

For the topping:

4 oz. chocolate chips, sugar-free

Steps:

1. Layer baking paper on a 6-inch baking pan and set to the side.
2. On low/medium heat, melt the chocolate chips in a saucepan.
3. Use a food processor on high to whip the almond flour and butter.

4. Add the peanut butter, Swerve and vanilla extract to combine fully.

5. Use a rubber scraper to smooth out in the prepped pan and empty the melted chocolate on top.

6. Cool in the refrigerator for 2 hours. Slice and enjoy!

Tricks and Tips:

- If you leave in the refrigerator, the flavors will become richer and the sugar will not be so granulated.

Chapter 6: Mousse Recipes

Avocado Mousse

Total Prep& Cooking Time: 35 minutes

Makes: 6 Mousses

Calories: 57

Net Carbs: 1.3 grams

Protein: 1 gram

Fat: 5 grams

What you need:

1 large avocado, shelled

3 tsp. lime juice

1 tsp. vanilla extract, sugar-free

1/4 cup sweetener, confectioner

3 tsp. agar agar

1 tsp. green tea powder

3 tbsp. cold water

Steps:

1. In a regular dish, dispense the water over the agar agar. Allow the mixture soak for 5 minutes before heating in the microwave for 1 minute on the medium/high setting.
2. Using a food processor with an S-blade, stir the avocado, sweetener, green tea powder, and vanilla extract until creamy.
3. Add the agar agar and lime juice to the mousse and stir well.

4. Taste test at this point to add more sweetener to your preference.
5. Spoon the mousse into a pastry bag and pipe into dessert dishes.
6. Cool them for 30 minutes in the refrigerator and serve.

Tricks and Tips:

- If you want variety, you can top the mousse with balsamic vinegar or mixed berries of your choice.

- Don´t have a piping bag in your kitchen? You can alternatively use a gallon sized ziplock bag. Just add the whipped cream and cut one corner of the bottom to the size you prefer.

Caramel Sea Salt Mousse

Total Prep& Cooking Time: 1 hour

Makes: 1 Mousse

Protein: 27 grams

Net Carbs: 5 grams

Fat: 26 grams

Calories: 368

What you need:

4 tbsp. water

1.6 oz. meal replacement shake mix, salted caramel flavor

2 tbsp. dark chocolate, unsweetened and chopped

1/4 cup heavy whipping cream

Steps:

1. In a food processor on high, whisk the heavy whipping cream for 4 minutes.
2. In a serving cup, mix the water and shake mix until combined. Add the whipped cream.
3. Spoon the mousse into a pastry bag and pipe into a glass or serving dish.
4. Put the glass in the freezer for 40 minutes, stirring the mousse about every 10 minutes.
5. Remove from the freezer and top with chopped chocolate before enjoying.

Tricks and Tips:

- Don´t have a piping bag in your kitchen? You can alternatively use a gallon sized ziplock bag. Just add the whipped cream and cut one corner of the bottom to the size you prefer.

Chocolate Mousse

Total Prep& Cooking Time: 10 minutes

Makes: 4 Mousses

Protein: 5 grams

Net Carbs: 4 grams

Fat: 26 grams

Calories: 268

What you need:

1 tsp. vanilla extract, sugar-free

4 tbsp. sweetener, confectioner

1 cup heavy whipping cream

4 tbsp. cocoa powder, unsweetened and sifted

1/4 tsp. salt

Steps:

1. Using a food processor on high, whisk the heavy whipping cream for 4 minutes.
2. Combine the sweetener and salt into the mixture. Then add the cocoa powder and vanilla extract until thickened.
3. Spoon the mousse into a pastry bag and pipe into serving dishes.
4. Serve and enjoy!

Tricks and Tips:

- Don´t have a piping bag in your kitchen? You can alternatively use a gallon sized ziplock bag. Just add the whipped cream and cut one corner of the bottom to the size you prefer.

- If you want a lighter mousse, simply beat 3 egg whites for 4 minutes in a food processor and fold in before spooning into serving dishes.

Lemon Cheesecake Mousse

Total Prep & Cooking Time: 1 hour 10 minutes

Makes: 5 Mousses

Protein: 3 grams

Net Carbs: 2 grams

Fat: 27 grams

Calories: 269

What you need:

4 oz. of heavy whipping cream

1/2 tsp. liquid Stevia, lemon flavored

8 oz. cream cheese

1/8 tsp. salt

4 tbsp. lemon juice

Steps:

1. Using a food processor on high, whisk the heavy whipping cream for 4 minutes.
2. In a dish, whip the cream cheese and lemon juice with an electric blender.
3. Add the mixture to the food processor and whip on high for 2 additional minutes.
4. Taste test the mousse and add more sweetener to taste.
5. Spoon the mousse into a pastry bag and pipe into serving glasses.
6. Dust the tops with lemon zest and cool in the refrigerator for 1 hour before serving.

Tricks and Tips:

- Don't have a piping bag in your kitchen? You can alternatively use a gallon sized ziplock bag. Just add the whipped cream and cut one corner of the bottom to the size you prefer.

- Thinking about using an alternative sweetener because of the aftertaste? Try it first as the lemon will overpower any trace of it.

Mocha Mousse

Total Prep & Cooking Time: 2 hours 25 minutes

Makes: 6 Mousses

Protein: 4 grams

Net Carbs: 4 grams

Fat: 39 grams

Calories: 389

What you need:

8 oz. mascarpone cheese, softened

3 tbsp. sweetener, confectioner

1 1/2 cups heavy whipping cream

2 tsp. espresso powder, instant

1/4 tsp. salt

3 tbsp. cocoa powder, unsweetened

1 tsp. vanilla extract, sugar-free

Steps:

1. In a food processor on high, whip mascarpone cheese and heavy whipping cream for 6 minutes.
2. Blend the cocoa powder and sweetener and pulse for a minute.
3. Finally add the salt, espresso powder, and vanilla extract until creamy.
4. Spoon the mousse into a pastry bag and pipe into serving cups or dishes.
5. Refrigerate for 2 hours before serving.

Tricks and Tips:

- Don´t have a piping bag in your kitchen? You can alternatively use a gallon sized ziplock bag. Just add the whipped cream and cut one corner of the bottom to the size you prefer.

Peanut Butter Mousse

Total Prep & Cooking Time: 10 minutes

Makes: 8 Mousses

Protein: 8 grams

Net Carbs: 5 grams

Fat: 34 grams

Calories: 369

What you need:

For the mousse:

1 cup Swerve sweetener, granulated

3/4 cup peanut butter

2 tsp. vanilla extract, sugar-free

8 oz. cream cheese, softened

2 tbsp. heavy whipping cream

For the whipped cream:

1 cup heavy whipping cream

3 tsp. Swerve sweetener, granulated

1 tsp. vanilla extract, sugar-free

Steps:

1. In a big dish, whisk the sweetener and vanilla extract using an electrical blender.

2. Add and whisk the peanut butter, heavy whipping cream, and cream cheese and mix thoroughly until creamy.

3. For the whipped cream, use a food processor on high to whisk the heavy whipping cream, vanilla extract, and sweetener for 3 minutes.

4. Add the peanut butter mixture to the whipped cream in small amounts.

5. Spoon the mousse into a pastry bag.

6. Pipe into serving glasses and enjoy.

Tricks and Tips:

- Don´t have a piping bag in your kitchen? You can alternatively use a gallon sized ziplock bag. Just add the whipped cream and cut one corner of the bottom to the size you prefer.

- The consistency will be creamier if you serve straight away. If you want a thicker mousse, place in the fridge for 4 hours and then serve.

- You can use this recipe to make peanut butter ice cream as well. Just transfer to serving size freezer safe containers and put into the freezer overnight. Pull out of the freezer about 10 minutes to let it soften before serving.

- Top with your favorite treats such as sugar-free fudge sauce or unsweetened chocolate chips.

Pumpkin Cheesecake Mousse

Total Prep & Cooking Time: 1 hour 25 minutes

Makes: 10 Mousses

Protein: 3 grams

Net Carbs: 2 grams

Fat: 18 grams

Calories: 215

What you need:

3/4 cup heavy whipping cream

15 oz. pumpkin puree, unsweetened

2 tbsp. pumpkin pie spice

12 oz. cream cheese, softened

2 tsp. vanilla extract, sugar-free

1/2 cup sweetener, confectioner

Steps:

1. Using a food processor set on high, whisk the pumpkin puree and cream cheese for 5 minutes.
2. Combine the heavy whipping cream, pumpkin pie spice, vanilla extract, and sweetener until creamy.
3. Spoon the mousse into a pastry bag and pipe into serving cups.
4. Refrigerate for 1 hour before serving.

Tricks and Tips:

- Don´t have a piping bag in your kitchen? You can alternatively use a gallon sized ziplock bag. Just add the whipped cream and cut one corner of the bottom to the size you prefer.

Strawberry & Blueberry Mousse

Total Prep& Cooking Time: 10 minutes

Makes: 6 Mousses

Protein: 3 grams

Net Carbs: 3 grams

Fat: 27 grams

Calories: 260

What you need:

8 oz. mascarpone cheese, softened

1/4 cup sweetener, granulated

8 oz. strawberries, sliced

1 cup heavy whipping cream

8 oz. blueberries, whole

3/4 tsp. vanilla extract, sugar-free

Steps:

1. Using a food processor set on high, whisk the mascarpone cheese and sweetener for 3 minutes until a smooth consistency.
2. Add in the heavy whipping cream and vanilla extract and continue to whisk for 2 additional minutes.
3. Spoon the mousse into glass cups, layering in the strawberries and blueberries and serve.

Chapter 7: Frozen Dessert Recipes

Cheesecake Bites

Total Prep & Cooking Time: 1 hour 10 minutes

Makes: 15 Bites

Protein: 1 gram

Net Carbs: 0.5 grams

Fat: 10 grams

Calories: 91

What you need:

1/2 cup sweetener, granulated

4 oz. butter, softened

1/2 tsp. vanilla extract, sugar-free

8 oz. cream cheese, softened

Steps:

1. Use a mini cupcake pan and line with baking cups. Set to the side.
2. In a stand mixer on high, cream the sweetener and butter for approximately 3 minutes.
3. Blend the vanilla extract and cream cheese until incorporated.
4. Spoon the mixture into the baking cups and freeze for 1 hour until firm.
5. No need to wait for them to defrost. Serve and enjoy!

Chocolate Chip Balls

Total Prep & Cooking Time: 1 hour 10 minutes

Makes: 16 Balls

Protein: 2 grams

Net Carbs: 2.4 grams

Fat: 6 grams

Calories: 80

What you need:

4 tbsp. cocoa powder, unsweetened

1/2 cup sweetener, granulated

4oz. butter, unsalted and softened

8oz. cream cheese, softened

1/4 cup chocolate chips, unsweetened

4 tbsp. cup water

Steps:

1. Using baking paper or a non-stick mat, cover a cooking sheet and set to the side.

2. In a food blender set on medium, cream the water and cocoa powder for 3 minutes.

3. Combine the sweetener, cream cheese, and butter. Turn the setting for the food processor to high and whisk for 4 additional minutes.

4. Use a rubber scraper to blend in the unsweetened chocolate chips.

5. Measure out the batter with a 1-inch cookie scoop and drop on the prepared cookie sheet.
6. The balls need to be frozen for 1 hour.
7. Remove from the freezer 10 minutes before serving.

Tricks and Tips:

- If there are any leftovers, simply place them in a freezer safe container for up to a week.

Chocolate Whips

Total Prep & Cooking Time: 1 hour 20 minutes

Makes: 12 Swirls

Protein: 0 grams

Net Carbs: 1.5 grams

Fat: 8 grams

Calories: 70

What you need:

2 1/2 tbsp. Swerve sweetener, granulated

1/2 tsp. vanilla extract, sugar-free

3 tbsp. cocoa powder, unsweetened

8 tbsp. heavy whipping cream

1/8 tsp. salt

Steps:

1. Set a cookie sheet out and layer with baking paper.
2. In a stand mixer on high, whip the sweetener and vanilla extract for 60 seconds.
3. Blend the heavy whipping cream, salt and cocoa powder for 3 additional minutes.
4. Scoop the whipped cream into a piping bag with a 1M nozzle.
5. Squeeze the contents on the prepared cookie sheet, creating individual swirls that look like ice cream on a cone.
6. Freeze for a minimum of 1 hour until firm and serve.

Tricks and Tips:

- You can get creative with this recipe and try out other flavors. Simply substitute 1 teaspoon of flavored extract in place of the cocoa powder.
- Don´t have a piping bag in your kitchen? You can alternatively use a gallon sized ziplock bag. Just add the whipped cream and cut one corner of the bottom to the size you prefer.
- If you prefer soft serve ice cream, simply let the whips defrost for approximately 10 minutes before serving.
- These can be frozen for up to 2 months in a freezer safe container, but we do not think they will last that long!

Coconut Bars

Total Prep & Cooking Time: 40 minutes

Makes: 14 Bars

Protein: 4 grams

Net Carbs: 4 grams

Fat: 20 grams

Calories: 213

What you need:

1 large scoop protein powder, vanilla flavored

4 oz. dark chocolate chips, unsweetened

1 cup coconut, flaked

3/4 cup coconut oil, melted

1 1/2 cups macadamia nuts, raw

Steps:

1. Using an 8-inch pan, cover with baking paper or a non-stick mat.
2. In a food blender set to high, blend the macadamia nuts and coconut oil until evenly mixed.
3. Combine the protein powder, chocolate chips, and coconut until mixed thoroughly.
4. Transfer the batter to the prepped pan and freeze for half an hour.
5. After it's set, slice into 14 individual bars.
6. Thaw for 10 minutes before serving.

Tricks and Tips:

- You can use other nuts in this recipe instead of macadamia. Experiment with cashews, walnuts, almonds or a mix.

Frozen Yogurt

Total Prep & Cooking Time: 1 hour

Makes: 8 Scoops

Protein: 3 grams

Net Carbs: 2.7 grams

Fat: 11 grams

Calories: 122

What you need:

3 cups plain yogurt, full fat and chilled

1 tbsp. MCT oil

2 tsp. vanilla extract, sugar-free

1 tbsp. lemon juice

4 tbsp. monk fruit sweetener, confectioner

8 tsp. blueberry syrup, sugar-free (optional)

Steps:

1. In a food blender set on medium, blend the lemon juice, MCT oil, and sweetener for 2 minutes until incorporated.
2. Add the yogurt and vanilla extract and stir in with a rubber scraper.
3. Place the bowl in the freezer for half an hour.
4. Once set, top with the blueberry syrup, if you prefer, and serve.

Tricks and Tips:

- This recipe is for soft serve yogurt. If you would like it to be harder, leave in the freezer for 6 hours before serving.

Key Lime Pie

Total Prep & Cooking Time: 4 hours 30 minutes

Makes: 6 Pies

Protein: 2 grams

Net Carbs: 2.8 grams

Fat: 21 grams

Calories: 219

What you need:

3 tsp. sweetener, granulated

1/2 cup pecans, raw and finely chopped

3 tsp. butter, unsalted

1/2 cup heavy whipping cream

3 tbsp. lime juice

1/4 cup sweetener, confectioner

2 tbsp. sweetener, confectioner and separate

4 oz. cream cheese, softened

1/4 tsp. salt

6 lime slices

Steps:

1. Set out a cupcake pan and line with baker or non-stick cups.
2. In a food blender set on medium, whip the cream cheese, lime juice, and 1/4 cup confectioner sweetener until creamed.
3. In a regular sized dish, combine and mix the remaining 2 tablespoons of confectioner sweetener and heavy whipping cream for 3 minutes.

4. Combine the whipped cream and cream cheese mixture using a rubber scraper.

5. Heat a small saucepan and melt the butter, sweetener, and pecans for 6 minutes. Stir in the salt and remove from heat.

6. Transfer the lime mixture to the cupcake cups and top with pecans.

7. Freeze for 4 hours to set. Remove the paper liner before serving.

Tricks and Tips:

- If the pies freeze for longer than 6 hours, remove from the freezer 30 minutes before serving.

Raspberry Ice Cream

Total Prep & Cooking Time: 10 minutes

Makes: 5 Dishes

Protein: 1 gram

Net Carbs: 3 grams

Fat: 16 grams

Calories: 183

What you need:

2 cups raspberries, frozen

1/3 cup sweetener, confectioner

1 cup heavy whipping cream

Steps:

1. Using a food processor on high, whisk the heavy whipping cream for 4 minutes.
2. Combine the raspberries and sweetener and puree for 2 additional minutes.
3. Taste test to ensure the sweetness is to your preference. Add 1 – 2 tablespoons of sweetener, if required and stir again.
4. Spoon into serving dishes and enjoy!

Tricks and Tips:

- You can add whatever frozen berries or fruit that you prefer to this recipe. Keep in mind that the berries will be the lowest in sugar.

- This is a soft-serve version of ice cream. If you want a harder version, you can use an ice cream maker, which will make the recipe more of a sorbet texture or simply freeze until the firmness you desire.

Yogurt Popsicles

Total Prep & Cooking Time: 1 hour

Makes: 12 Popsicles

Protein: 1 gram

Net Carbs: 5 grams

Fat: 6 grams

Calories: 80

What you need:

1 tsp. vanilla extract, sugar-free

8 oz. mango, diced

1 cup Greek yogurt

8 oz. strawberries, diced

1/2 cup heavy whipping cream

Steps:

1. In a food processor set on high, whip the yogurt until fluffy.
2. Blend the strawberries, vanilla extract, mango and heavy whipping cream until smooth.
3. Transfer to popsicle molds and freeze for 2 hours.

Tricks and Tips:

- This recipe will also make soft serve ice cream that can be served after mixing the ingredients. There is no need to freeze.

Index for the Recipes

Chapter 5: Tart and Bar Recipes

Tart Recipes:

Butter Tarts

Blueberry Lemon Tarts

Fruit & Cheese Tarts

Hazelnut Tart

Bar Recipes:

Chocolate Fudge Bars

Granola Bars

Peanut Butter Chocolate Bars

Strawberry Rhubarb Bars

Chapter 6: Mousse Recipes

Avocado Mousse

Caramel Sea Salt Mousse

Chocolate Mousse

Lemon Cheesecake Mousse

Mocha Mousse

Peanut Butter Mousse

Pumpkin Cheesecake Mousse

Strawberry & Blueberry Mousse

Chapter 6: Frozen Dessert Recipes

Cheesecake Bites

Chocolate Chip Balls

Chocolate Whips

Coconut Bars

Frozen Yogurt

Key Lime Pie

Raspberry Ice Cream

Yogurt Popsicles

Made in the USA
Middletown, DE
29 September 2019